A KETO DIET

TABLE OF CONTENT

CHAPTER -5

BENEFITS AND EXPECTATIONS OF A KETOGENIC DIET

CHAPTER -6

SUCCESS TIPS FOR BEING ON A KETOGENIC DIET

CHAPTER -7

LOSING AND MAINTAINING WEIGHT ON A KETOGENIC DIET

CHAPTER -8

FREQUENTLY ASKED QUESTIONS

CHAPTER- 1

WHAT IS A KETO OR KETOGENIC DIET?

A keto diet or a ketogenic diet is a diet which emphasizes on utilization and break down of fats for the energy sources of the body to help achieve weight loss and to provide diet therapy in many diseases, but most commonly to suppress seizures.

A typical ketogenic diet is high in total fat, moderate in protein and low in carbohydrates. Among the three energy giving nutrients, it stresses on utilizing fats as a basic source of energy. This diet encourages the process of ketosis through increased fat metabolism. A regular diet is high in carbohydrates, moderate in protein and low in fat.

In a ketogenic diet, 60-80 % of the total calories needed for energy come through fats. This diet has been gaining popularity for weight reduction recently. Initially in the 1920s it was mainly used to provide diet therapy to young patients of epilepsy. Many children who were suffering from seizures had reported to respond positively to this kind of diet and fasting and had reported less incidences of seizure attacks as compared to the ones not taking this diet. Constipation and unpalatable nature of the diet for these kids were the main problems reported. Medium Chain Triglycerides found in abundance in coconut oil was specifically noted for its beneficial properties for such patients.

Its unique metabolic properties has been claimed to be adopted to treat many diseases as well as to reduce weight in a non-traditional way. A ketogenic diet also known as a keto diet is not a well-balanced diet, therefore dietary supplementation and fiber is needed to be taken along with this diet to make it more balanced. Many people who have tried to achieve health benefits through this kind of diet have found its unique properties and have gained set goals. There have been many positive sides as it helps in catabolizing and breaking down fat deposits in the body. Many benefits have been reported for weight reduction, seizure controlling, improving glycemic index and many more. Still many aspects of this diet need in-depth study and research to fully understand the limitations and boundaries and to fully understand its benefits in many chronic diseases.

To avoid food nutrient deficiencies to occur, nutritional supplements and fiber needed to be added if one is planning to adhere to this kind of diet for a long period of time. In this diet calories from protein and carbohydrates are replaced by calories from fat. Each gram of protein and carbohydrates provide four calories while each gram of fats provides nine calories because fats and foods containing fats are dense in calories, therefore more satiety is achieved by eating less. This diet is dense in calories but deficient in most nutrients, consequently supplementation is needed. The lacking nutrients are necessary to be taken in the form of supplements to avoid deficiency diseases to surface.

During digestive process, carbohydrates enter in the blood stream in the form of glucose. All the extra amount of glucose not wanted for immediate energy need is stored in the form of glycogen in the liver and muscle tissues by the help of a hormone released by the pancreas called insulin. Whenever the blood glucose level rises insulin is released from the pancreas which helps in glycogen synthesis and storage in the liver, muscle tissues and very small amount in the brain and white blood cells. This process is again reversible whenever the need of glucose arises and blood glucose level goes down.

Whenever the blood glucose level goes down the normal range and is not replaced by the diet, this stored glycogen is readily available and converts into glucose and enters in the blood stream maintaining the normal level through a hormone also released by the pancreas called glucagon. Glucagon plays an opposite role of insulin and breaks down the stored glycogen and converts it again to glucose to maintain blood glucose level. The natural system goes on automatically as long as the natural cravings for each food needs are met.

Our brain prefers to use glucose as a form of energy in the presence of glucose. During fasting when all glucose stores are empty or in ketosis, our brain learns to adapt the prevailing conditions and starts utilizing the alternative energy available through fats or break down of fats. Whenever the glycogen storage in the liver gets depleted either by insufficient dietary intake of glucose or inadequate synthesis of glycogen due to lack or absence of insulin, the process of ketogenesis or synthesis of ketone bodies take place. The presence of these ketone bodies causes ketosis which can also be a result of fasting, starvation as well as direct consequences of taking a ketogenic diet.

Ketogenic diet promotes breakdown and utilization of fats for energy and discourages utilization of carbohydrates as a source of energy. Protein in this diet is just enough to maintain growth and repair required in the body. Due to the absence of glycogen stores as a result of low carbohydrates diet, the liver starts to metabolize fats instead to furnish energy. This is promoted by ketogenic diet but can happen naturally during long starvation, stress and fasting conditions. Exercise also supports and helps in this.

Through a ketogenic diet, four parts of total energy requirement comes through fats and only one part is divided between both proteins and carbohydrates. Recipes needed to be developed to make things easier for patients and people who wish to try this diet regimen. What food items can be used liberally, what are moderately restricted and what are strictly restricted. A detailed list of these needed to be provided to them so that they can create their own recipes. Recipe development is an art that does not require much effort. Each individual is different from the other and each one has different activity factor. Each diet needed to be individualized accordingly taking into consideration height, weight, activity factor, likes, dislikes, tolerances, intolerances, preferences, allergies, etc.

Health professionals have been found to be concerned about the proper guidance that needed to be provided to these people. How to start on this diet and what can one expect out of it? How to control and deal with ketosis and how to check serum and urine ketone level? Increasing activity and dealing with the symptoms and whatever needed for proper management. A proper guideline is needed to mentally prepare them of the expectations, tips, benefits and maintenance needed. What needed to be eaten and what needed to be avoided. How to create more palatable recipes? How to sweeten your meal without regular sugar? How to keep oneself motivated and strong? How to have patience and will power? When to exercise and how much is enough?

Many benefits that have been reported are facts that cannot be ignored. Most important benefit that it helps in the breakdown of built in fats and helps in catabolizing adipose tissues cannot be ignored. Adipose tissues are stubborn and are hard to break down. Exercise and increased physical activity do help in breaking down built in fat deposits. Eating a well-balanced diet but with long time intervals also helps in catabolizing fat deposits and can create a situation close to ketosis. Ketogenic diet helps in mobilizing fats to burn up for energy and brain adapts to utilize the energy of fat substrates i.e. ketone bodies. Excess of ketone bodies can get excreted through urine, sweating, breathing and increased physical activity.

Ketosis does also play a protein sparing role. In the presence of ketones, body will not breakdown muscle tissues for the supply of glucose as a source of energy, instead it will utilize the energy from ketones. Body will prefer ketones over glucose and therefore protein would not be oxidized to produce glucose. In normal conditions, whenever blood glucose level goes down and glucose and glycogen supplies are not available, proteins are metabolized to maintain blood glucose level within normal ranges.

In the absence of carbohydrates there are more breakdowns of fats and the body gets adapted to utilizing fats and fat stores in the body instead of relying solely on glucose. As the amount of carbohydrates is lessened in the diet and the stores of glucose and glycogen gets depleted, the insulin level automatically goes down. This causes lipolysis or breakdown of fat and fatty acids leading to ketosis. Our brain in normal conditions consumes around 20% of our total energy output. It prefers to utilize glucose over any other source of energy.

In the absence of carbohydrates, body starts to breakdown muscle tissues to furnish energy needed immediately. Amino acids of protein can be catabolized to provide glucose whenever needed in the absence of carbohydrates. To prevent the process of catabolism and breakdown of muscle tissues during weight reduction and to encourage anabolism or synthesis of muscle tissues and to encourage catabolism or breakdown of adipose tissues or fatty tissues, a diet promoting ketosis is suggested. Ketosis allows the body to get adapted to utilize fats instead of proteins and carbohydrates. Careful planning is needed to bring out the best results needed.

In order to divert body's attention towards utilization of fat stores in the body and to spare proteins for muscle synthesis, a high fat, low carbohydrate and moderate protein diet is suggested. Ketogenic diet needs to be followed after taking into consideration the medical condition of any given individual. It is comparatively a new phenomenon and trend towards weight reduction as historically it has been associated with and used practically to overcome symptoms of epilepsy. More and more claims started to appear for its benefits for many problematic conditions and diseases. It has been found to be beneficial for killing cancer cells, improving glycemic index, found beneficial in type 2 diabetes, controlling seizures, and so on.

More solid studies are needed in this regards to benefit the general public from many therapeutic effects. Awareness programs for understanding the true nature of the diet are needed. Periodic health checks are needed when using this diet practically. Professional supervision and its importance also cannot be ignored. To avoid any kind of danger that might be associated with this, one needs to understand the matter in depth and proper utilization of professional help and guidance whenever and where ever needed. Preparing one-self mentally and knowing why this is suggested, how to go along with it, what are the pre-requisites, what are the limitations and benefits and how it actually works. Deep understanding of the nature of the whole program is looked-for. What one can expect out of it, what tips are desirable, where to look for motivation and help and so on.

Many people due to being handicapped or due to immobile can go for this option. Conditions in which increasing the physical activity or exercise are not advisable or practical, the option of ketogenic diet can work wonders. It should be the last resort not the first one and should never be adopted just for trial and error efforts because switching over diets can be risky. Professional guidance is of real concern here. Preparing oneself emotionally would benefit and help in passing through this phase successfully. One should go back and resume normal diet as soon as possible or after successfully passing through this phase and achieving their dietary goals. Normal diet does not mean over loading your diet with carbohydrates especially simple sugars. Abstinence from alcoholic and carbonated drink is advisable for all.

Ketogenic diet and fasting produces same kind of results. During fasting, a balanced diet necessary to be taken at long intervals. In a ketogenic diet, 3-

4 small meals of therapeutic diet plan needed to be followed on a daily basis. It has been suggested by relevant studies that weight reduction does happen through ketogenic diet but mostly it reappears after switching to normal routine once the set goal has been achieved. This has been proved wrong if you stick with the right choices and good habits. Following a ketogenic diet, achieving the good results and then going back again on old habits cannot help. Keeping oneself strong towards good changes and adapting them for life long will show better and long lasting results.

CHAPTER -2

FOODS ALLOWED AND RESTRICTED IN A KETOGENIC DIET.

What foods needed to be eaten and what foods needed to be avoided when following a ketogenic diet requires understanding of the three basic energy giving nutrients known as the macro nutrients. The only energy giving nutrients among the six major nutrients include carbohydrates, proteins and fats which constitute a major bulk of our daily diet. Both proteins and carbohydrates provide same number of calories per gram i. e. four calories. Fats being dense in calories furnish nine calories per gram.

In order to understand what foods are needed to be eaten and what foods are needed to be avoided in a ketogenic diet, good understanding of food sources of fats, carbohydrates and protein is necessary. Following given list helps in determining the food sources of fats, proteins and carbohydrates.

Food Sources Of Fats

Excellent food sources of fats include butter, margarine, oils, ghee, full cream, lard, mayonnaise, etc.

Good sources of fat include full cream milk, full cream yogurt, prawns, lobster, organ meat, bones broth, lamb, beef, mutton, poultry with skin, eggs, full cream cheese, etc. These food sources are also rich in good quality protein and are poor sources of carbohydrates except milk and milk products which contain lactose sugar.

Significant sources of fats containing foods are also rich in carbohydrates. These include dry fruits, nuts, seeds, avocado, etc.

Food Sources of Protein

Excellent food sources of protein include egg, mutton, beef, fish, lamb, prawns, lobster, poultry, cheese, yogurt, milk, etc.

Good food sources of protein include pulses, beans, tofu, chickpeas, gram, nuts, seeds, gelatin, etc.

Significant sources of protein include corn, rice, wheat, barley, etc.

Poor sources of protein include cucumber, all leafy green vegetables, citrus fruits, yellow squash, radish, mushrooms, onion, turnips, avocado, green pepper, brussels sprouts, beet root, eggplant, lemon, okra, capsicum, zucchini, garlic, pumpkin, cabbage, tomatoes cauliflower, carrots, asparagus, bean sprouts, broccoli, etc.

Food Sources of Carbohydrate

Excellent food sources of carbohydrates include common sugar, fructose or fruit sugar, honey, brown sugar, molasses, hard candies, etc.

Good food sources of carbohydrates include starchy vegetables and fruits, bananas, potatoes, sweet potatoes, peas, beans, gram, chickpeas, rice, wheat, barley, sorghum, millet, corn, mango, cheeko, etc.

Fair sources of carbohydrates include milk and milk products, green leafy vegetables, non-starchy vegetables, butter squash, avocado, tomatoes, cucumber, ice berg, cabbage, green pepper, zucchini, Brussels sprouts, eggplant, lemon, pumpkin, asparagus, carrots, cauliflower, capsicum, onion, bean sprouts, turnips, mushroom, garlic, radish, beet root, okra, etc.

List of Food items that can be used to create recipes for a ketogenic diet include the following.

Ketogenic Diet

To create recipes for a ketogenic diet, it require techniques of mixing foods with each other with limited choices in such a way that their palatability is increased and individual needs are met. This needs pure challenging situation and very good planning. A ketogenic diet promotes the excess usage of fats and fat rich sources of foods therefore these diets must be rich in butter, cream, ghee, margarine, olive oil, coconut cream, peanut butter, canola oil, palm oil, sesame oil, macadamia, coconut butter, flax seed oil, lard, avocado oil, creamy salad dressings, mayonnaise, butter cream frosting, cream cheese, coconut oil, etc. Fat selection should be according to individual tolerance and intolerance, likes and dislike and preferences. Any fat which is found to be intolerable must be replaced by other fats and oils. Olive oil, coconut oil, coconut cream and avocado oil is advisable for their therapeutic properties.

As ketogenic diet is low in carbohydrates, low carbohydrate vegetables can be used in good combination and different seasonings and methods of cooking can be applied to create and develop mouth-watering dishes and recipes. Vegetables that can be used include avocado, spinach, lettuce, fresh cilantro, fresh mint, parsley, cabbage, fresh basil, ice berg, summer squash, Brussels sprouts, cauliflower, green pepper, zucchini, black olives, mushrooms, and fair amount of carbohydrates from the list of fair sources of carbohydrates can be used.

A ketogenic diet is moderate in protein so moderate amount of excellent sources of protein must be included. Good sources and significant sources of protein needed to be avoided as they are good sources of carbohydrates as well and basic idea behind a ketogenic diet is to have a diet that is low in carbohydrates to promote ketosis and break down and utilization of fats in the body. Beef, poultry, fish, prawns, lobster, organ meat, mutton, cheese, yogurt, egg, lamb, etc. can be used in moderation and in combination with different low carbohydrate vegetables to increase and improve palatability of the diet. Each individual likes and dislikes needed to be given due consideration as well as food tolerances and intolerances. Fattier cuts of meat and chicken with skin needed to be used where ever possible.

Different ways of cooking e. g. baking, stewing, barbecuing, frying, steaming, can be used to make food more likable and palatable. Different combinations of color to improve garnishing can make food more appealing and improves its acceptability. Different herbs and spices can be used to improve the flavor of foods e. g. basil, parsley, ginger powder, garlic powder, black pepper, cinnamon powder, etc. Use of various available sauces and flavor enhancers to develop creative recipes can be pure fun e. g. tomato ketchup, soy sauce, Worcestershire sauce, mustard sauce, barbeque sauce, etc.

As ketogenic diet being low in carbohydrates it does not allow the usage of corn or other flours to be used as thickening agents. Instead we can use the alternatives available. Coconut flour, cream cheese, whipped cream, heavy-cream, gelatin-powder, macadamia nuts-flour, almond flour, pecans flour, coconut cream, peanut butter, coconut butter, etc. can all help in making gravies, soups and sauces that could be used in good combinations for better results.

In a ketogenic diet energy should mostly come through 60-80 % fats, 15-25% protein and 5-15 % carbohydrates. Total carbohydrate intake should be less than 60 grams. Protein intake could vary between 1-2 gm. for each kilogram of body weight. Rest of the energy should come through fats. Around 20-25 gm. of fiber should be added daily to make up for a low carbohydrates diet and consequently low fiber diet. Flax seed can be incorporated into various recipes for its high fiber content. Salads with rich dressings can be helpful in furnishing of more fiber and increasing the fat content of salads. Multivitamin supplements needed to be taken regularly.

CHAPTER -3

REACHING KETOSIS THROUGH KETOGENIC DIET

Whenever our liver is short of energy from carbohydrates, it starts metabolizing fats for energy as an alternative source. During the catabolism or break down of fats to furnish energy ketone bodies are produced which causes ketosis. Ketosis always occurs inside our body whenever our body is deficient of energy from carbohydrate sources but can also happen due to some medical problem and because of taking a ketogenic diet. During the process of lipolysis breakdown of fats occur and triglycerides are broken down to provide three molecules of fatty acid chains and one molecule of glycerol.

The fatty acids produced by this process can be utilized by our body as a secondary source of energy in the absence of glucose. Breakdown of fats and fatty acids are promoted by fasting, exercising or increased physical activity, starvation and ketogenic diet. The body physically gets to start adapting to utilizing the fats. Fat stored in our body in the form of adipose tissues, is being metabolized to furnish energy to the body. The breakdown of fatty tissues in our body helps us in saving our muscle tissues. Weight is being lost at the expense of the built in fats and not at the expense of built in muscles. Increased physical activity, fasting, starvation and ketogenic diet all are beneficial in achieving this to some extent.

The utilizing of fats instead of carbohydrates results in the production of ketone bodies and the state of ketosis. Our liver is responsible for the synthesis of ketone bodies. Ketone bodies are important because our brain which consumes around 20 % of all our energy need prefers glucose over any other available energy source. But in the absence of glucose it is unable to utilize long chain fatty acids as they are bound with albumin protein and are unable to furnish energy to the brain. These ketone bodies produced can be utilized by the brain for energy.

Our brain consumes high amount of energy as compared to the amount of mass it possess and we cannot even blame it as it never sleeps. Even when we are fast asleep, our brain keeps functioning and helps us to digest the food that we have eaten, circulate all the blood around our body and keep all internal functions to work automatically without our involvement and any effort. So the brain does deserve lots of energy that it needs.

Ketone bodies are acidic in nature and therefore excess of these in our blood can be harmful for people who are suffering from diabetes and needs treatment to overcome ketoacidosis which could lead to diabetic coma and even death. A normal healthy body is capable of handling this and maintaining the blood pH level within normal ranges. Ketoacidosis can happen mostly in type I diabetes but can also happen in type II diabetes cases rarely. Excess of ketones in the blood and urine for a long period of time can damage internal organ e. g. kidneys and liver. Therefore extra water needed to be taken in order to flush out these through urine, breath and sweating and to free the body of its toxicity. Water also helps in diluting these.

Signs of Ketosis and its testing

Excess ketone bodies produced during stress, starvation, fasting or a ketogenic diet can start accumulating in the blood stream causing typical fruity odor in breath and passing out extra ketones in the urine. A urine sample can be tested to find out and evaluate the presence of ketone bodies in urine at home level using specific strips needed.

Following are some of the reported signs and symptoms associated with ketosis.

- Presence of ketone bodies in urine.
- Fruity odor in breath.
- Extra thirst.
- Head ache, fatigue and tiredness.
- Frequent urination.
- High energy level and clear thinking.
- Weakness and dizziness.
- Stomach ache, nausea, and sleep problems.

- Unusual taste in mouth.
- Cold feet and hand.

Ketosis is not a harmful condition for a healthy human being and through ketogenic diet it is used to maximize the breakdown of stored fat in the body. Initial stage of reaching ketosis can be disturbing and may be a cause for discomfort but the signs and symptoms start to subside as the body gets adapted to the new energy sources. Urine sample may not always show the presence of ketone bodies and can be misleading. Excess intake of water or utilization of ketones during increased physical activity can be the causes for misleading urine sample. Drinking extra water may dilute the urine to give wrong report.

A person going through ketosis may find it to be an unpleasant experience due to the body's reaction and also due to the unpalatable nature of the diet. Very high levels of ketones needed to be avoided as they can have damaging effects on the liver and kidneys and therefore can be toxic. Extra ketones can be removed by drinking extra water, breathing it out through lungs and using it up by increasing the physical activity.

CHAPTER 4

KETOGENIC DIET FOR DIABETICS

Diabetes is a chronic disease in which the metabolism of carbohydrates is affected due to inefficiency or total failure of pancreas to produce insulin or resistance of body cells to insulin. There are three types of diabetes.

In type I diabetes also known as juvenile or insulin dependent diabetes, insulin is needed to be injected with intervals as pancreas are totally unable to produce this. This type of diabetes is controlled through insulin injections, diet and exercise.

In type II diabetes the body is able to produce insulin but the cells of the body are resistant to it.

Therefore patients are treated through hypoglycemic drugs, diet and exercise. These patients may at times need doses of insulin to control blood sugar.

Type III diabetes occur during pregnancy and could be controlled by diet and exercise. Around one in five may need to take hypoglycemic agents.

A ketogenic diet can be allowed to be followed by patients suffering from diabetes under controlled conditions and proper guidance and supervision of professionals concerned. Ketoacidosis is a serious condition in which a diabetic patient can develop signs and symptoms of diabetic coma which could be life threatening if proper medical care is not provided in a timely manner.

A normal healthy body is capable of maintaining the pH of the blood. People who are suffering from diabetes are incapable of reversing ketoacidosis and need external medical intervention. Over nutrition is also one of the causes of diabetes and eating in limitation is very important to avoid obesity leading to many chronic diseases.

Diabetic ketoacidosis and its symptoms sometime may appear within a day. Signs and symptoms may include loss of appetite, abdominal pain, confusion, weakness, shortness of breath, nausea, fatigue, vomiting, dry skin, excessive thirst, dry mouth, low blood pressure, fruity smell in breath, difficulty in breathing, excessive urination, etc. Testing the blood for sugar level and urine for ketone level can confirm the signs and let the person suffering know when to consult a physician. At times emergency care may be needed to avoid coma or even death. These patients might require insulin, rehydration and electrolyte intake.

CHAPTER -5

BENEFITS AND EXPECTATIONS OF A KETOGENIC DIET

Before starting a ketogonic diet one need to get aware of what to expect while passing through this phase practically for its benefits. How it could benefit and preparing mentally to handle the initial time period specially those who feel carbohydrates are inseparable part of their lives is very important. A ketogenic diet is all about changing a way of how you eat your diet. Initial time period can be rough till the body gets adapted to the new diet regimen.

Its beneficial effects for patients suffering from epilepsy are well known. This diet has been found to be lessening the attacks of seizures and in many cases eliminating seizures.

Keeping the blood glucose levels low and ketones level high have been found to be beneficial for cancer patients as it has been reported to kill cancer cells.

Many people suffering from type II diabetes have experienced better control over blood glucose level and feel there are many benefits attached to it.

Decreased level of joint pain, controlled blood pressure, and lessening of heart burn are few other reported benefits.

Weight loss through reduction in adipose tissues instead of muscle tissues is one more known advantage.

Other known benefits which still need more studies and evidence include Alzheimer's, Parkinson's, narcolepsy, brain trauma, amyotrophic lateral sclerosis, acne, brain cancer, polycystic ovarian syndrome, etc.

The transition time period from normal diet to ketogenic diet lasts for few days when the body gets adapted to a new primary source of energy i. e. fats can cause few disturbing symptoms. These symptoms may include headache, irritability, fatigue, weakness and most of these symptoms may subside within a week or so. The serum, urine and breath ketone level will increase. Long term usage may affect your serum lipid profile which could even be positive. Serum lipid profile and blood glucose level needed to be checked at least once a month to keep them within normal ranges.

In the beginning within two weeks of ketogenic diet, dramatic weight loss may occur due to depleted stores of glycogen from liver and muscle tissues consequently loss of water held by these cells. Total water loss will be proportional to the total muscle mass. Ketogenic diet has been gaining popularity since last twenty years for weight loss and its therapeutic properties for many chronic diseases.

While following a ketogenic diet, serum ketone level must not cross the borderline and therefore needs regular checking. Increased blood acidity could have damaging effect on the liver and kidneys.

A ketogenic diet has been found to be especially beneficial for brain functions and treatment of brain diseases. It has historically been proven to eliminate or decrease seizures. Our brain contains high amount of fats as compared to other organs and therefore consume high energy as well.

Adaptation to this diet may take from one week to twelve weeks. A person may pass through the phase of fat phobia once adjusted fully to this diet.

CHAPTER -6

SUCCESS TIPS FOR BEING ON A KETOGENIC DIET

Increase physical activity

Increasing physical activity in addition to following a diet regimen will help in losing weight even faster and helping in developing muscle tissues. Half an hour of brisk walking, cycling, swimming or jogging all are beneficial.

Increase intake of fluids

Increasing water and fluid intake can help in excreting extra load of ketone bodies and relieving the body of toxic waste especially in hot weather conditions when there is increased physical activity and consequently increased sweating.

Decrease intake of alcohol

Alcoholic drinks also contribute to energy so must be discontinued and they can also cause carbohydrate overload.

Be more creative with recipes, keep your spirits high, avoid caffeinated drinks, keep yourself motivated, keep a check on urine and blood ketone level which needed to be maintained, keep a track of weight loss, understand and adhere to the diet protocol, etc.

If sticking to a regular or standard ketogenic diet is difficult, one can try a cyclical ketogenic diet. In this one need to follow a ketogenic diet from Monday to Friday and on weekends it is allowed to take a carbohydrates overload. In this exercise is needed on weekdays only and can rest on weekends and have carbohydrates overload and stores for the whole week on weekends. If cyclical ketogenic diet is not suitable then one can go for targeted ketogenic diet. In targeted ketogenic diet 25-50 gm. of carbohydrate is allowed before a work out.

Good understanding of what is needed to be eaten and what needed to be avoided is very important. Keeping vigilant to various signs and symptoms of any kind of health problem or concern should not be ignored.

CHAPTER -7

LOSING AND MAINTAINING WEIGHT ON A KETOGENIC DIET

Losing and maintaining weight on a ketogenic diet is very important and one need to keep oneself motivated towards it for life long results. How many calories a person will need on a keto diet will depend primarily on individual height, weight and activity factor and on the fact of calorie input and calorie output. One pound of weight is lost when we take 3500 calories less in the diet than we utilize it e.g. if some ones calorie intake is 1200 and calorie output is 1700 then this person will lose one lb. per week if he sticks on taking 500 calories less for one whole week. In order to increase your intake you have to first start catabolizing more which can be achieved by increasing physical activity.

Regular brisk walk, swimming, cycling or any form of aerobic exercise need to be part of daily routine. Your daily energy expenditure will depend on your metabolic rate. Your metabolic rate is high when you are active and it slows down when you are sedentary. Lessening the use of machinery in our daily lives to accomplish various tasks, and making better use of our own efforts which could be easily achieved through little exertion all can have beneficial response towards increased physical activity at our own home level. In this way you do not have to spend extra time, effort or money to leave your home and visit a gym. Light to moderate activity could be achieved through this way which is required initially. Later on when your body gets fully adapted to the new diet then you can plan for more active and vigorous exercises and may schedule your gym visits on regular basis close to your neighborhood.

How much body fat you must lose will depend on the percentage of existing fat in your body of your total body weight. Increasing physical activity in addition to following a strict ketogenic diet regimen will give more beneficial and long lasting results. Losing faith, spirit and motivation during initial difficult time period will only leave you in the middle of nowhere.

Correct understanding of suitable ratio of macro nutrients needed is essential. Good understanding of good, fair and poor sources of macronutrients is required. 50 gm. of carbohydrates can easily be consumed in a minute in the form of a candy. The same amount of carbohydrates can be distributed in the whole day in the form of high fiber non starchy vegetables. Protein intake can also vary according to individual height and weight and activity factor. During increased physical activity or vigorous exercising you may be able to consume a more liberal intake of good quality protein as these will be utilized for muscle anabolism.

One can start from 50 % of calories from fats. Watch for one week and let the body get adapted to high fat content. Choose only those fats which you feel your body tolerates well. Fats can be consumed easily if incorporated in soups or emulsions. Emulsions can be prepared using nut flours. Drinking lots of broth prepared from bones will help in reducing dehydration and any deficiency of sodium. Addition of little lemon juice will help in preventing potassium deficiency.

Rest and sleep is of utmost importance during following a ketogenic diet. It helps in keeping the body in good working condition especially when we have started a new diet altogether. Pay more attention to your body and needs of your body. Respond to its need whenever needed. If you feel thirsty do not ignore. Ketones can cause toxicity and can have damaging effect if you do not drink enough water or fluids needed. These toxins like others needed to be relieved through urine so you stay healthy. So drink water whenever you feel thirsty.

First week on a ketogenic diet may be difficult so be prepared for it from the beginning. This is temporary because your body is passing through an adaptation phase. You have introduced a fat diet to it and it is trying to adjust to it. One very important thing to remember is not to cheat. Please do not cheat yourself. It will not help you in any way as the whole system will get disrupted. During ketogenic diet the blood sugar level need to remain at lower levels and carbohydrates are not the only culprits to raise sugar level. Proteins are made up of amino acids and these can convert to glucose to maintain blood sugar level. Fats can also contribute to this. Glycerol a metabolite of fats can turn into glucose.

This diet has been found to be helpful for mental alertness and improved mental capabilities. Patiens play an important part in this diet because weight loss can be slow and steady. Rapid weight loss is never good and therefore should not be our goal. Weight loss may vary from person to person depending upon their genetic makeup, body metabolic rate, physical-activity, sleeping pattern and food ingestion. Each individual is unique in his makeup and individual response to this diet will also be unique.

From the beginning till around three weeks into this diet people may find it difficult to exercise. For these three weeks light exercise is recommended. Later on the intensity of exercise may be increased. Keeping your insulin level low will help you in breaking down built in fat and will discourage anabolism of fatty tissues. Keep checking your weight on weekly or fortnightly basis. Make a target goal where you want to reach. Calculate your ideal body weight for your height. For 5 feet, 100 lbs. for females and 106lbs. for males are ideal. With one inch increase in height we have to add 5lbs. for females and 6lbs. for males. For each inch of extra height, keep on adding the pounds. Ten percent above or below the ideal will also come within the ideal. Any variance more than this or less than this will be considered overweight or underweight. If someone is more than 20 % of his ideal body weight he will come under obese category.

Do not eat when you are not hungry but only when you feel hungry. Be patient and avoid artificial sweeteners as much as possible. Sleep more and do not take unnecessary stress. Proceed wisely with your diet therapy. Avoid alcoholic drinks and fruits. Instead take fibers, minerals and vitamin supplement. Increase physical activity smartly. High fat content of ketogenic diet will help in suppressing your hunger you need not force feed yourself. There is lot of built in energy inside your body which need to be burnt. Let that energy take care of the energy needed by the body.

According to one authentic study people burn more energy on low carbohydrate diet while resting. Rest and sleep helps the body to get adjusted to things easily.

Measure your waist circumference on weekly basis. It is also advisable to keep a track of your blood pressure and serum lipid profile once a month or once in two months.

You may lose 1-6 pounds during the first week and 1 pound on weekly basis after the first week. But this may vary with individual cases. Maintaining your weight will require you to change your eating habits and lifestyle. Following most of the rules of healthy living, eating and adapting may have far reaching implications that may prove to improve overall health.

There are three types of ketogenic diet standard ketogenic diet, cyclic ketogenic diet and targeted kitogenic diet. A standard ketogenic diet does not allow any overload of carbohydrates. A person can be active as much as possible but it has been a known fact that people keep losing weight on this diet even if they do not feel they have enough stamina for exercising and if they do not exercise. In cyclical ketogenic diet a person can do work out twice or thrice a week during the week days and is allowed a load of carbohydrates during the weekend. During weekend a person can take rest and no need for any exercise. In targeted ketogenic diet a person can work out during the week and before working out he is given 25-50 gm. of carbohydrates load for stamina.

This diet is famous among people who are either unable to exercise or people who do not like to work out. It is a known fact that this diet work wonders even without exercising and the results are more long lasting as it deals with the base line of dealing with the problem of wrong kind of fat deposits inside the body. It helps in reducing these built in hulks and attacks them with a purpose. It has been looked all around by professionals for its safety and till now has been declared to be safe enough to be practiced. Keeping a check on ketone levels, drinking enough water, resting and sleeping well, increasing activity whenever easily possible and sticking with the diet regimen will help and bear fruitful results. Keeping your patience intent and not letting it go and keeping self-motivated will help.

Do not keep a check on your weight on daily basis and do not measure your waistline every now and then. Ketogenic diet is not magic and will take its time to bring good and fruitful results. Get support from people around and talk out your problem and discuss with people who have tried this diet. Pay more attention on your interests and less on thinking about food and do not think about foods you are not allowed to eat. Once you get tempted and eat out of your diet pattern you may come out of ketosis and it will take few days for you to get back again to ketosis. Whenever you are tempted to eat something sweet and feel you are having a sweet tooth then select foods which are prepared by using artificial sweeteners e. g. diet jelly, etc. just to curb the temptation.

CHAPTER -8

FREQUENTLY ASKED QUESTIONS

Q.   Are all low carbohydrate diets ketogenic diets?

A.   No, not all low carbohydrate diets are ketogenic diets.

Q.   What is a ketogenic diet?

A. A ketogenic diet promotes the utilization of fat energy over protein or carbohydrate energy.

Q. How does it work to benefit?

A. It emphasizes on the catabolism or break-down of adipose-tissues rather than muscle-tissues.

Q. Is it safe to use?

A. It has been tried and tested and for a healthy individual it does not pose any health risks.

Q. Do we have to take it through-out our life time?

A. You need to stick to it till your ideal weight to height or set-goals have been achieved.

Q. Is it safe in all conditions?

A. No, it is not safe in all conditions. It is not advisable to pursue this diet in chronic liver or kidney disease. Also, it is not safe during pregnancy and lactation.

Q. Can I reduce weight through this diet?

A. Yes, this diet is suitable for weight reduction.

Q. How do we distinguish this diet from other diets?

A. This diet is high in fats, adequate in proteins and low in carbohydrates.

Q. In how many days do we achieve ketosis?

A. In around two days' time.

Q. Can I increase physical activity along with this diet?

A. Yes, exercise along with ketogenic diet is advisable.